THE STRATEGIC WATER STRIKE

A GUIDE TO LOSING WEIGHT THE HEALTHY WAY

BY FRANK TREVINO

Love Sick Dog Publishing/Corpus Christi, TX

Love Sick Dog Publishing. Copyright 2008 by Frank Trevino. All rights reserved. Printed in the United States of America. No part of this book may be reproduced or transmitted in any form or by any means, electronic or mechanical, including photocopying, recording, or by any information storage and retrieval system, without written permission from the publisher. For information, address Love Sick Dog Publishing at ftrevino44@yahoo.com

Visit Myspace.com/lovesickdogrecords
And
Myspace.com/thestrategicwaterstrike

Library of Congress Cataloging-in-Publication Data applied for
ISBN 1440435839

FIRST EDITION

This book is dedicated to my wife, Elizabeth.

ACKNOWLEDGMENTS

The following people helped me greatly in writing this book. They are in no particular order:
Elizabeth Budd, Valorie Sanchez, Edie Stovall, Cornelia Valdez, and Colton Taylor

A Special Thank You to Mom, Mr. and Mrs. Budd, and all my family and friends

Some people want money, but all I want is change.
-Love Sick Dog Publishing

Contents

Foreword

As a 5'7" and 135 lb. sixteen year old kid growing up in Corpus Christi, I was always disappointed about how much my ribs showed; all the while a six pack glistened in the sun. What I wouldn't give to go back in time and slap that kid. You see, back then I always wanted to be a bit heavier, but nature always has its usual way of making you realize you really don't know what you have until you get too much of it.

I still remember a time I was standing next to my high school track coach. He was talking to an old friend who came in from out of state. His friend who happened to be a bit muscular, yet a bit round in the waist said, "I guess it's the South Texas heat that keeps you all so thin." I kind of shrugged my shoulders and said, "I guess." I was a little envious because I could not put on weight as easily as he did, but I didn't realize he was probably thinking he should be a little lighter. I didn't understand it wasn't just the Texas heat that was keeping me from gaining weight. It was my metabolism and also that I was continuously exercising. If I wasn't playing high school football, then I was running track.

It wasn't until I was in my thirties that my metabolism started to slow down and I started quickly gaining weight. My weight went up to 168 lbs., but I really didn't care. After all, 168 lbs. isn't bad, right? Yet, it seemed that the more people I talked to the more I found people were concerned about their own personal weight. I would hear other people talk to each other about weight loss; and if someone said that he or she had lost weight, then there would be an enthusiastic, "How did you do it?" However, there was never a definitive answer on how to do it exactly without being hungry.

I wasn't concerned about losing weight, but I was concerned that I was always feeling tired and worn down. I then started to drink more water to see if it would help. And it did, but I also started to lose weight without trying to. After I lost weight, more and more people kept telling me how thin I was looking. They started asking how I did it, and I didn't know. It wasn't until I really started to think about what I was doing that I then discovered the Strategic Water Strike.

When you hear a song that touches you, sometimes you think that's what you wanted to say, but you couldn't really explain the joy or the hurt you were feeling. Being a songwriter and owner of Love Sick Dog Records I've written many songs, but I never thought of writing a weight loss book. Why would I? I've been 135 lbs and under, half of my life. Still, I decided to write this book because so many people have wanted to know how exactly to lose weight without feeling as though they are starving themselves. And, I think I can explain it.

Is There a Doctor in the House?

No. So, why would you take weight loss advice from someone who is not a doctor? After all, I am just a regular Joe. Well, our grandparents weren't doctors (for most of us, anyway), but they still gave us good advice; didn't they? The point is most good advice is given to us by someone who has experienced it. And, the experience I had with this diet helped me to lose 25 pounds. Besides, this plan is cheaper than most prescribed diets, I'll try to keep it simple, and this method in losing weight really does work. Period! Actually, there is a little secret I should mention; but don't tell anyone. All diets work, theoretically, of course. The one little problem is how to fight the huge craving for food. Well, that's the one predicament this book addresses.

Most diet books tell you what small portions to eat and try to convince you to hang on to whatever willpower you have left after a long day's work. They don't tell you how to control your hunger. They leave out the biggest detail. What do you do if you are still hungry after you have eaten the prescribed microscopic portions? They don't address the basic tools of knowledge to help fight the craving for food. **This book doesn't tell you what exactly to eat. It teaches you how to suppress hunger using the Strategic Water Strike Method.** The Strategic Water Strike Method is a technique that can be used with any diet. The main objective is to utilize water at the right moment during your meals. This will help you eat a reasonable proportioned meal so you can still have your cake and eat it too. Part of the problem is that if you don't eat the food you love, you'll probably stop dieting. Who wants to eat rice cakes the rest of their life? I don't. I refuse to live life that way. The struggle is to find a balance between healthy food and food you like. This technique is meant to help bridge the gap between dieting and eating your favorite food by limiting the amount of food you eat.

But do not misunderstand me; you can't have all the cake you can eat. You still have to eat healthier. The Strategic Water Strike method is meant to minimize the amount of food you eat, but you still need to use good judgment on what to eat. This practice is meant to give your stomach the opportunity to be at the point where it can calmly say, "I've had enough. I can stop eating." As opposed to it screaming, "I am starving! Give me everything on the menu!" (Fun fact: At one time you could have ordered everything on the Taco Bell menu and a diet soda for under $40.)

Drinking more water is not uncommon weight loss advice and neither is counting calories or exercising, which I mention later in this book. The Water Strike method is unique because it utilizes water before and after meals to naturally suppress hunger. This enables you to not only survive on smaller portions of your favorite food, but also thrive.

Nip It in the Bud

As the great comedian Don Knotts used to say, "Andy, you got to nip it in the bud!" That's right. To be successful in any diet you have to get off to a good start. It's following through with the commitment part that gives us problems. But every single choice plays a big part in continuing a diet. Commitment is one choice at a time. So, the first choice is to decide if this is really what you want to do.

Don't read this book until you have made a decision to change! Once you have decided to change your eating habits, use the Water Strike and commit to it because as I mentioned in the previous chapter, all diets work. If you are going to continue reading the rest of this book, then hopefully you have already made up your mind to make a change in your eating behavior. Using the Water Strike method will help with that change. However, before trying the Water Strike, realize healthy eating starts one choice at a time at restaurants and grocery stores. You have to make your decision to lose weight not at the point of eating, but at the point of purchase.

For example, TGIF, Apple Bee's, and Chili's have items listed on their menus with the amount of calories in them. The selections are limited, but you still have a choice. On the other hand, if you frequent the Olive Garden, then you won't know how many calories you are eating. The Olive Garden does not list any calories on the menu. (And believe me; they don't want you to know.) You won't always be able to eat at restaurants that have calories listed on the menu, but try to frequent the ones that do.

Furthermore, if you are going to continue to eat at restaurants and fast food places that do not offer better choices (some fast food places now offer apples shaped as fries), then you won't be eating healthier or be able to lose much weight. But you should at least look at each company's website to know if they offer any healthy choices. Many companies list the amount of calories each item has on their respective websites.

Use the same discretion when you grocery shop. Make smart choices by reading the labels to know what ingredients are in the foods you are buying. The Water Strike helps you to eat less. But if you have foods that have a high amount of fat in your kitchen, then you are going to eat them. And if that is the case, then you have failed yourself not when you eat them, but when you bought them.

Reading the labels on products helps you to make healthy purchases. But sometimes it becomes complicated because you may have to decide between fat, sugar, and sodium. And, that decision is not an easy one. The majority of products have either too much sugar or fat. Most of the time I would rather have the sugar because there is a chance to burn it off before it turns to fat. Fat, on the other hand, is much harder to lose. (If you are diabetic or have any other medical conditions, then you should consult your doctor.) In certain situations a little fat may be better than a lot of sugar, so it may not always be easy to choose. If you do find yourself making a difficult decision on which is better, just know you are on the right track because you are at least aware of what is on the label.

Moving forward, you must make a decision to lose weight by making better choices or just put this book down. If you constantly make bad choices, then the Water Strike method will not help you lose weight. No diet will for that matter. You have to make better choices from the point of purchase, or you will not be successful at losing weight. Again, I'm not saying that you can't have chocolate cake and ice cream. I'm just saying that you can't have a triple cheese burger and have cake and ice cream for dessert. But you can have a balanced meal, and then eat a reasonable portion of cake and ice cream.

In later chapters, I discuss some of the other choices to make in your diet; but I would like to reiterate, you don't have to give up all your favorite foods. Just have them in moderation. I would also like to stress that Water Strike Method is not a quick fix to weight loss. Using this technique should result in gradual healthy weight loss. The Water Strike method helps to cut calories so you can enjoy some of your favorite foods and still lose weight. With a new outlook on the point of purchase, and a few modifications to the ingredients and food in your diet, you can achieve your weight goals. So, if you have made your decision to start dieting by making smarter choices, the next chapter describes how to curb hunger using the Water Strike method.

Chalk It Up to Science

As a kid, I remember touring the local museum and seeing a picture of a dinosaur in a swamp. I was told the dinosaur lived in the swamp because it was able to get all the nutrition it needed from there. I later learned the real truth was dinosaurs could not live in a swamp because their body weight would sink their footing so deep into the ground that they couldn't move. Shocked! How could science pull the wool over the eyes of poor unsuspecting Dino loving kids? Well, junk science is unfortunately still around with every other diet book telling you the opposite of what was considered good to eat. Eggs were once considered good for you, and then all of a sudden they weren't. Are eggs better for you now? I just can't tell you. But I can tell you what is and what will always be true. A good balanced meal is healthy for you; and yes, you can eat eggs.

The trick to healthy weight loss with a balanced meal is to utilize water. With most of the Earth covered with water and most of the human body comprised of it, it should make sense that water would be a major key to our diet and health. However, too often we mistake thirst for hunger. That's right. Most of us are thirsty when we think we are hungry. Did you ever wonder why you can't just eat one salty potato chip? It's because the chips actually make you thirsty. But since you think you are hungry, you continue eating chip after chip. If this ever happens to you, reach for a glass of water.

Great…so you paid money for this book and all I have to say is to drink more water? Yes, but strike when the iron is hot. It's the timing that helps curb hunger. The Strategic Water Strike utilizes the drinking of water right before meals. This will help to distinguish between hunger and thirst. Rule out thirst disguised as hunger by drinking water first. This technique will help you realize many times you actually aren't very hungry, and it will mentally condition you to break with old eating habits.

Drinking eight glasses of water sporadically throughout the day will help keep you hydrated; but it doesn't help curb the feeling of being hungry when it's time for breakfast, lunch, or dinner. If you drink water between meals just to have your eight glasses of water, then you are wasting the opportunities that help manage your appetite.

The Strategic Water Strike method uses the recommended eight glasses a day to help control over eating during meals. It helps to rationally decide how much cake and ice cream you really want to eat, or if you want them at all. It will help you to eat slower so you can savor the taste of your favorite food. Many times we are prevented from enjoying a meal because the food goes through our mouths very quickly. Our taste buds don't get a chance to actually taste anything. The food goes by like a passing race car. We get a glimpse of the car, but we really don't get a good view. Then, we eat two or three times more than we should just to find out what we are missing.

The Strategic Water Strike method was developed with the premise that weight loss can be achieved by eating food you love. And that's not just once a day. It's eating three meals a day with snacking in between them. How do you lose weight by eating food you like? Do it by slowing down your eating pace to savor food. This helps you enjoy a smaller portion. You don't have to eat large amounts of food to enjoy them. **You can actually enjoy your favorite foods more by eating less.** Use the six steps in the Strategic Water Strike method to slow your eating pace down and enjoy food.

1. **Drink two eight ounce glasses of water**. Before you eat anything…and I mean anything! Drink two eight ounce glasses of water before each of your three meals a day. You will then notice that your hunger drops significantly. The reason for the two glasses of water is psychological. It is easier to drink two smaller eight ounce glasses of water than to drink one 16 ounce glass.

2. **Eat a small appetizer.** Eat something like a piece of fruit, a serving of yogurt, a salad, a few low fat chips (not the whole bag), or something healthyish. Remember, part of this strategy is to include healthy choices, so choose wisely. This step is usually for a larger meal like dinner. Some people are not big breakfast eaters, so this step is optional for smaller meals. If you are a big breakfast eater, then this would apply. Personally, I try to eat an apple once a day before one of my meals because of the fiber it provides, and because I like apples. Choose something that's healthy, but something that you like.

3. **Start eating**. Depending on how the water affects you, you may then opt to start eating your main course. The water will help in portion control as you serve your meal. If you feel like you are so full of water that you are unable to eat, then you may elect to wait a few more minutes. You may even want to wait 15 to 30 minutes. Do not force yourself to eat; but do eat at some point.

4. **Let your food settle**. After you have eaten a part of your meal, let's say half, then stop and let your food settle. (That just means wait a few minutes.) The reason for this is it gives your stomach time to decide how much more you can eat. If only you were like the gas pump that shuts off when the fuel tank is filled. Unfortunately, you aren't. By the time you realize you're full, it's too late - the last piece of pizza has already been eaten. It's like eating a food grenade. Instead of waiting for the first one to go off, another is eaten. Then, you wonder why your stomach aches. Learn to let food settle. Take a pause during meals to realize how far up the fuel gage has gone. It will take a few minutes for you to realize how much more you should eat. As your food meets up with the water you just drank, the food will absorb the water, then expand. I don't know if it's the expansion of the food, or just the weight of water and food that gives your stomach the signal that you are getting full; but it receives the signal nonetheless.

5. **Finish your meal.** At this point take advantage of the drop in hunger. Remember, you are using this technique to cut back on calories; so use this opportunity to realize how many more calories to cut from your diet. **This method should teach you to eat for taste and not for hunger.** If you are used to eating larger portions, then you should have a substantial amount left over.

6. **Leave room for another eight ounce glass of water.** If you are unable to drink another glass of water after your meal, then you might have over eaten just a bit. But depending on how many calories you want to cut out of your meals, the third glass is meant to keep you from over eating. This step may be optional depending on how full you feel. If you are not a big breakfast eater and skip step two, then a third glass of water during breakfast may not be necessary.

Well, I know what you are thinking. That's a lot of water! And, that doesn't include that you may want to drink something with your meal. If you choose to drink something with your meals, which most people do, then try to limit what you drink to eight ounces. This will also help to cut out calories because you will be drinking fewer calories. A twenty-four ounce drink that might have 360 calories can be reduced to eight ounces and 120 calories.

Let's now go through some scenarios of the third glass of water.

Scenario 1: If you drink two glasses of water and schedule yourself to only eat 600 calories in a meal, but still feel hungry, then by all means drink the third glass of water to help stop your hunger.

Scenario 2: If you drink two glasses of water and eat your meal and feel you don't need the third yet, then you can wait awhile to drink it. You may wait to drink it until you start feeling hungry again; but don't wait too long or the third glass won't have any effect.

Scenario 3: If you drink two glasses of water and are finished with dinner and don't think you need a third glass of water, then don't drink the third glass. Dinner is the hardest to judge if the third glass of water is needed. If you wait too long to decide to drink the third glass before bed, then the notorious midnight snack craving might creep up on you. The third glass of water will probably kill the midnight snack craving, but it might also keep you up at night going to the bathroom. If you have a very early dinner, you may choose to have another snack later and even a fourth glass of water.

The method also varies if you exercise a lot. If you do, then drink a bit more water throughout the day just to replenish all the fluids lost from working out. Also, the average person will feel partially full after two glass of water. If you are a very large person and hunger isn't curbed at all after two glasses, then try three eight ounce glasses of water before each meal. Don't be afraid to drink water. Some reports even suggest dividing your weight by two and using that number for the amount of ounces to drink each day. Example: 150 lbs. divided by two is 75 lbs. That would be 75 ounces of water a day as opposed to only 64 ounces.

Use the Water Strike method with every meal. This technique is meant to curb hunger by assuring you don't mistake thirst for hunger. Don't over eat then drink water! The water is intended to prevent over eating. You do not want to end up like the guy who was in a pancake eating contest. Afterwards, he drank lots of milk which the pancakes then absorbed. He swelled up like a balloon and had to get his stomach pumped. Don't be that guy!

It's the Simple Math That Will Fail You

An important thing to know about this method and all diets is not to lose count of your calorie intake because the same basic principle still applies; you have to burn more calories than you eat to lose weight. (If you are going to refuse counting calories, then you might want to skip this chapter altogether.)

A recent study showed that people who actually wrote down what they ate were more likely to lose weight. I think the reason they were more likely to lose weight is because they knew how many calories were in the food they ate. They probably also stayed away from places like a buffet, where they couldn't count calories or judge how much is one serving size.

Now, you're not going to have to keep track of every single calorie you will ever eat. But as you get started, it's important to count every calorie because this will help to calculate how many calories you are essentially burning. As you continue to count calories and see results, you will eventually become comfortable with what you feel you can and cannot eat; but for now, count calories to help figure out where all the extra calories are coming from. It may be from drinking too many sodas or cups of coffee during the day; or it may be from eating too many servings of chips, or eating candy bars in between meals. However, you won't know until you start keeping count.

The First Week

In the first week you decide to start this diet, you're going to keep track of all your calories and weigh yourself at just the beginning and at the end of the week. If you don't usually exercise, then don't start exercising during the first week you have started the Water Strike method. You want to find out the average amount of calories you naturally burn each week. If you start to exercise, then that will increase the amount of calories you burn. You want to find out what's the lowest amount of calories burned. (Wow! That's unusual. There's a diet book telling you not to exercise?)

If you do exercise regularly, then continue exercising as long as you understand if you stop exercising you will have to recalculate the amount of calories that you burn.

At the end of week one you will have reached one of the following three results:

1. Weight loss – if you lost weight, then you burned more calories than you ate.
2. Weight gain – if you gained weight, then you ate more calories than you burned.
3. Same Weight – if you stayed the same, then you ate the same amount of calories you burned.

This may seem like a "tell me something that I don't know" moment; but it's an important one because the results will tell you how many calories you actually burned in the first week…..that's if you kept count of all your calories.

The X factor in this equation has always been not knowing how many calories you are burning. But by keeping track of all your calories in the first week, you can find out. And, that will help you plan how many calories to eat in each meal. The next examples will explain how to do that; so pay close attention to this part.

Example one: If your weight is stable from week to week, and you average eating 2,600 calories a day, then you are burning the exact amount of calories that you are eating. If you want to lose weight, then you can start losing one pound a week by just eating 2,100 calories a day. Lose 500 calories a day, and you will lose one pound a week.

This is crucial because now you don't have to starve yourself to lose weight.

Now you know that for each pound you want to lose a week, you have to cut back 500 calories a day. And you can do that by using the Water Strike method to help control your hunger. You can plan how many calories to enjoy in meals instead of planning to skip lunch or dinner.

If this is the case, then you can eat 600 calories for breakfast, lunch, and dinner and still have 300 calories left over for snacking. If you eat only 400 calories for breakfast, then use the 200 left over calories for lunch or dinner or vice versa! Because you are drinking so much water, you may not be as hungry at some meals. If this is the case, then use the left over calories from one meal to help when you are hungrier during another meal, or to splurge on the sweets you were craving.

Example two: You lost one pound and averaged eating 2,100 calories a day.

If you lost just one pound in that week, then you burned an average of 2,600 calories a day in that week. Since you are eating 2,100 calories and burning 2,600, you are burning 500 calories more than you are eating. Just continue cutting out 500 calories a day and you will continue to lose weight.

The last example is a little more complex.

Example three: If you gained two pounds and averaged 3,600 calories a day, then you still burned 2,600 calories a day. However, if this is the case, then you need to cut 1,000 calories out of your meals a day just to stay at your current weight.

In the first example the magic number was 500 calories to cut every day to lose just one pound in a week. In the third example the magic number is still 500 calories, but it was in the wrong direction. For every 500 calories eaten extra a day, one pound was gained in the week. (2,600 calories burned a day plus 3,600 eaten day = 1,000 extra calories a day and two pounds a week.)

If you are still gaining weight, then you are not burning enough calories, and you need to cut back on food; or (gulp) start exercising. Remember if you decide to start exercising and burn 200 extra calories a day, you will only have to cut out 300 calories a day because the difference is still 500. (How do you know if you burned 200 calories? You won't until you track all your calories.) Also, after awhile you may stop losing weight because your body will adjust to your diet and exercise. This is commonly referred to as "Hitting the Wall." If this happens, then you will have to reevaluate your diet and exercise routine and recalculate how many calories you are eating and burning. As you lose weight, your body will start burning fewer calories.

Let me stress the importance of counting calories at this point. You need to count because this establishes what you can eat. If you are only burning 1,200 calories a day and you are eating 1,300, then you will become discouraged. You may feel like you are trying very hard, but are not seeing any results. Also, if you don't see any result, then you can take this information to your doctor. It may be that you have a problem with your glands, but check with your doctor first.

The Second Week and Everyday After

Weigh yourself daily from here after. Some critics say it is not good to weigh yourself daily because you don't want to become obsessed with it; but keep track daily to know which direction your weight is going. Do not expect big results daily, but do expect weekly results. Why waste seven whole days of dieting to find out you are going in the wrong direction? Weigh yourself everyday at the same time. The best time to be weighed is in the morning. Believe it or not, you lose weight during sleep. If you are able to have an early morning bowel movement, then that would be the optimum opportunity to get an accurate reading of what you weigh.

When you are getting your blood sugar tested, for example, it is recommend you fast before you get tested for the best results. If you eat, it will skew the results of your blood sugar test. The same principle is true for your weigh-in. You don't want those results skewed either because a pound or two can make a big difference in calculating how many calories to eat. Also, sodium plays a big part in getting an accurate reading. Make sure to limit sodium intake. Sodium can alter your weight by two to three pounds. It helps to have a scale that calculates body mass and water percentages. This will help in monitoring if weight was really gained, or if you are retaining water from consuming too much sodium.

During your daily weigh-in don't forget to weigh yourself with the same type of clothing. If you weigh yourself with only shorts and a shirt, then make sure to do that every time. Don't wear socks one time and not the other. Keep what you wear during your morning weigh-in consistent.

Even though you are going to weigh yourself daily, again, it's the week to week results that measure success or failure.

You still have to decide which foods are healthier and how many calories to eat. Using this water technique just helps control the craving for more food if you do decide to cut back on calories. The great thing about drinking water is it is one less thing you have to count. So, you can't lose count of it ever because it does not have any calories...Ever!

But really, the hardest part is to not lose track of your calorie intake. Don't put yourself in a losing position by not investigating the menus of the restaurants you frequent. Do a little research to find out what items to purchase and choose the lesser of two evils. You will be surprised how many times companies have tricked you into buying unhealthy items you thought were healthy. Some of those items may have been the worst things on the menu. Examples of such corporate shenanigans are:

1. **Serving a loaded salad**. Most places serve salads that are high in calories and fat. The salads are loaded with cheese, bacon, high fat salad dressing and other unhealthy toppings. Most salads are made with iceberg lettuce, which has almost no nutritional value. If you are going to eat a salad, then limit the toppings and eat it with dark leafy greens. Romaine lettuce and spinach have the most nutritional value. Also, watch out for dressing that contains high fat content and high fructose corn syrup. We will address high fructose corn syrup in the next chapter.

2. **Grilled is better**. In most cases it is not, and is sometimes the worst thing on the menu. Most of the time if it says grilled, then it is loaded with sodium and heavily marinated. Remember, a large amount of sodium will make you retain water, thus making it difficult for you to get an accurate weight reading.

3. **Serving size**. Some items advertised claim to be low fat or low in calories, but that depends on the serving size. Oreos are low fat if you just have one. Subway is also low in fat if you eat just one six inch sandwich; but eat a foot long sandwich, and you will be eating almost as many calories that are in a burger. (Also, eating a Subway with cheese and their dressings loads up on the fat. That's one thing the commercials fail to mention.) Eating at a buffet is not recommended because you can't really

judge the serving size. And when it comes to buffets, your eyes are usually bigger than your appetite. Besides, it's usually a waste of money because you won't be very hungry if you use the Water Strike Method.

The important thing to remember is you don't have to give up the items you love; you just have to have them in moderation. The Water Strike method will help you do that. After all, you are allowed 65gs of fat a day in a healthy 2,000 calorie diet; but the less fat the better. Do your research so you don't end up eating 65gs of fat and half of your 2,000 calories all in one meal with the grilled chicken and a salad that you thought was healthy.

Say No to the High Fructose

One of the worst mistakes to make during dieting is not to know what you are eating. All products are required to list the ingredients and nutrition they contain on their labels. Most of us are aware of where nutrition is listed on the label, but the ingredient information is usually in very small print. It's important to realize the ingredients are not listed in random order. Ingredients are listed by what is used most to make the product to what is used the least. There are many ingredients in foods that can either help or derail your dieting. The worst ingredient culprit is high fructose corn syrup.

Let's try to understand the harmful effects HFCS can have on your diet. I am going to concede the fact that HFCS tastes very good; I am not going to lie to you. It does. Given that, this mighty foe can still be defeated. What makes HFCS so dangerous is two fold.

First, HFCS numbs your body's ability to tell when you are full. So, you will still be hungry…or rather still feel like you are hungry after a heavy meal. The main focus of the Strategic Water Strike Method is to utilize water to control hunger, and eating HFCS will undermine your ability to do that.

In full disclosure, I am not a doctor or scientist. I do not have scientific data regarding high fructose corn syrup. The corn industry is disputing whether HFCS has negative effects, but let me give you an example of a personal experience I had in Boston. While on vacation there, I decided to put this theory to the test. I was in the Boston Market and decided to order a huge cheese steak sandwich. Under normal circumstances I wouldn't be able to finish it because I wasn't very hungry. But I ordered a large soda (which by the way has HFCS listed as the second ingredient). Needless to say, I ate the whole sandwich and could have eaten more. Where did it go? Well, I wasn't sitting next to Houdini, that's for sure. I believe it was the soda with the HFCS that made it possible, but don't take my word for it. Try your own experiment. Eat a meal you usually eat with a soda. Then try to eat it again the next day with the Strategic Water Strike Method. What do you have to lose…..except calories.

Second, HFCS is one of the hardest if not the hardest sugar to get rid of in your system. It turns into fat easier than other sugars. That means if you are exercising, then you'll have to work out longer. You'll have to eat even less to accomplish you weight goal. The old cliché of work smarter not harder applies here, so stay smart and avoid the HFCS.

Do your homework and read the labels. Look specifically for the words "High Fructose Corn Syrup". Many words describe sweeteners like sucrose and dextrose, but HFCS is public enemy number one. Avoid products listing HFCS high on the ingredient list. Do not underestimate the power and frequency of high fructose corn syrup; it lies where you may least expect it. It is in some ketchup and barbeque sauces and this will hinder your decision on how much you should eat. This ultimate Trojan horse can kill any diet, and it's in almost everything you buy. It's in soda, jelly, bread, and even in your favorite saltine crackers. Did you know it is in fat free salad dressing? Is that why eating just a salad is so unfulfilling? Do not let this ingredient sweet talk you into getting on your meals. I can not stress this enough. **It lies in your food and lies to your stomach**. If you read the label, and HFCS is anywhere near the top ingredient, do not eat it!

Besides drinking water, avoiding HFCS is one of the most important aspects to controlling hunger. You have to control hunger in order to manage your calorie intake. Constantly drinking and eating HFCS will undermine your control of hunger and your goal of healthy weight loss. So, look before you leap; or rather, look before you eat. You can eat most kinds of food in moderation; but you must **Say No to the High Fructose!**

Check the Obvious

Are you tired all the time? Are your lips chapped? Are you always sleepy? Do you have a lack of energy at certain times of the day? Does it take five cups of coffee just to get you through the morning? Then check the obvious. Maybe you're just dehydrated. Drinking eight to ten glasses of water a day has always been good advice, but doesn't it make sense that water is a key to health? Does the fact that most of Earth is covered by water or that your body's composition is comprised of water help you realize water serves a crucial part in your diet? Well, there are other things that should give you reason to rethink water as an important part of health. Why is it when some medicines are prescribed, they are to be taken with a glass of water? Most diet pills are directed to be taken three times a day with… Oh… a glass of water (not to mention the small print that reads, "With proper diet and exercise"). So, cut out the middle man and drink more water. Mind you, I am not telling you to stop your prescribed medications. After all, I am not a doctor. However, next time you don't feel quite right, or if you feel extremely hungry, check the obvious.

Like everything in life, too much of anything can kill you…even water. For example, there was a woman who died when she entered a radio contest. The contest winner would be the one who could drink the most water within a certain period of time. The woman died because her organs gave out from drinking over five gallons of water. Was it obvious dying could be possible from drinking too much water? No, it wasn't. So, the more water the better is not always true.

How do you know when you have had enough water? Are you in danger by drinking so much water? Should you drink tap or bottled water? These are good questions that deserve answers. Let us exam all of them.

First, your body needs water within days or you will die. But if you drink too much, the water will not only flush out toxins, but also important vitamins and minerals; so, how much is enough? A good way of monitoring yourself is to notice the color of your urine. If your urine is a dark yellow, then you haven't had enough. The dark color is all the waste your body is disposing. If it is colorless, then you have flushed out all your bodies waste for the day and you may be fully hydrated. Also, if your lips are chapped, then drink more water immediately. Chapped lips are a tell-tale sign you have not had enough water. Start drinking water and chapped lips go away.

Second, you are not in any danger by drinking a lot of water unless you drink a mass amount within a short period of time. You would have to drink many gallons, and your body won't let you do that unless you really force yourself. Remember, water naturally tells your body you are full.

If you spend a lot of time outdoors in extreme heat, you do need to drink extra water beyond the Water Strike Method just to stay hydrated. Drink a couple of extra glasses before you are exposed to extreme heat, or exercise to prevent dehydration. Most people don't realize they are dehydrated until it's too late. Another good rule is to measure your weight before and after any strenuous activity. For every pound you lose by sweating, drink one glass to get back to your normal hydrated self. You'll be surprised you could lose up to five pounds in a matter of hours after being in extreme situations.

Third, should you drink tap or bottled water? Well, it is a little more complicated than you would think. Although tap water is getting a reputation for not being as clean as it should be, bottled water is now being criticized for being in a plastic bottle and more expensive. That's right. Whoever you choose to talk to will give you a different answer.

On one hand, I have a friend who works for the water department and she won't drink tap water. But I drink tap water everyday and I don't feel any different. I guess it just depends on the kind of water that you are used to drinking. People always say that when in Mexico you should not drink the water; and they are right. Mexicans don't feel the effects of their own tap water because they drink it everyday and their bodies have adjusted to whatever bacteria are in it. The tap water in the United States is generally safe to drink, and it has fluoride in it. So, you might see an increase in cavities if you don't regularly drink tap water.

On the other hand, bottle water is supposed to be cleaner; but read the label to know where it is from. Some critics say that bottled water is just tap water that has been processed into a bottle. Companies advertise it's from a mountain spring, but that may not necessarily be true. Also, bottled water is more expensive than tap and comes in a plastic bottle that is not biodegradable.

The answer to tap or bottle is not a simple one, but which ever one you choose is the right one as long as you choose water.

Cookies for Breakfast

When we were young we were told what to eat and when to eat it. Do you remember someone telling you that you could not have cookies for breakfast? Do you remember how excited you were when you found out there was a cereal that had cookies in it? Cookie Crisp where have you been all my life?! What a great loophole. But somehow, now that we are older, we figured out no one is in charge to tell us how to live our lives. We forget about looking for loopholes and disregard the old eating principles. In most cases, we eat what we want when we want it. The inmates now run the insane asylum! Anyone care for a triple meat cheese burger?!

Maybe, it is all those years of being told to finish everything on our plates. That's probably what taught us that after a good meal our stomach should feel very heavy; but shouldn't we feel a little lighter? It's almost like we just want more. Is it our irrational fear that we won't have anything to eat later that we insist to eat all we can? And, we now have a perception that a real meal has to have something heavy in it, like meat. We forget it's not the type of food that makes us gain weight; it's the mass consumption of calories. We let down our guard when it comes to eating a salad with many fat filled toppings. Refocus on the basic principles of eating; watch what you eat.

Use the Water Strike method to change your perception of what to eat. Because the Water Strike helps curb hunger, you can eat lighter foods and still feel full at any time of the day. Traditional food doesn't have to be eaten at traditional times. Cereal, oatmeal, eggs, and pancakes can be eaten for breakfast, lunch, or dinner as long as you watch the calorie intake. Kellogg's Cereal had a successful advertising campaign with their Pinch an Inch slogan. It announced cereal is not just for breakfast any more and that you could lose weight by eating their cereal two out of three meals a day. Genius! (What a way to double or triple their sales!) But it's not just the low calorie cereal that helps lose weight, it's also the skim milk that cuts calories and makes you feel full. The point is, you can eat traditional breakfast foods for lunch or dinner, or vice versa; but make healthy choices.

The Water Strike method is not just a technique to curb hunger; it is a state of mind. It's a life style choice to decide not to let hunger control you. Take back control of hunger by rethinking what to eat. Don't limit the food you like to only a certain time of the day. Utilize healthy food you like at any meal and to help with snacking. Snacking between meals is important because it speeds up your metabolism; not eating slows it down. So, snack with your favorite healthy food. It is also important to snack because the hungrier you get, the more unreasonable you become in regards to portion size. Snacking helps preserve discipline when serving regular scheduled meals. If you do not snack between meals, then you will eat a lot more during meals. Use the Water Strike method and snacking to enjoy more of the things you like at any time of the day; but also use them to serve a smaller portion on your plate.

Why not have cereals or oatmeal for dinner? Why not have cookies for breakfast? That's not real food you say. Well, yes it is. It is very real food with very real calories.

Coke vs. Pepsi

Have you taken this soda challenge? Did you know it is not a multiple choice question? Nope. It's a trick question. The answer is of course water, but let me explain.

Water naturally quenches thirst and helps curb hunger, but drinking soda that contains high fructose corn syrup has the opposite effect. High fructose corn syrup numbs the senses that allow you to know when thirst is quenched or when you are full. That is why you can drink a few 12oz cans of soda and still feel thirsty. You assume the sodas will quench your thirst, but they never do. Yet, when it comes to water, you can barely stomach one eight ounce glass of water. The Coke vs. Pepsi Challenge is rigged; they are both losers. Any sodas that contain HFCS, like Coke and Pepsi, will minimize the effect of the Water Strike method because they increase your appetite.

Drinking sodas with HFCS will also kill your taste for water and fruit. That will make using the Water Strike method very difficult. The Water Strike method is not only about drinking water, it is also about making healthier choices like fruit. Try this challenge: Next time you are thirsty, drink a soda; then try drinking some water. The result may shock you. The water will taste so bad that you probably won't drink more than two sips. You'll get the same result if you drink soda before eating fruit. Try eating an apple and drinking a soda. The apple will taste bad no matter how much you love apples. The HFCS in the soda will win every time. If you continue to drink HFCS, then you will lose the small battles between healthy and unhealthy choices, and eventually lose the diet war.

Sodas that contain HFCS will also affect the amount of sweets and unhealthy foods you eat. If you eat a lot of sweets, try to notice what's on your tongue. Eating, but mostly drinking, HFCS will keep you from noticing a layer of sugar on your tongue from eating too many sweets. HFCS will also prevent you from noticing the layer of grease on the roof of your mouth after eating French fries or potato chips. The more HFCS you ingest, the less you will notice the tell-tale signs of controlling the things you should not be eating. Sodas that contain HFCS are the most counter productive to dieting because they betray your taste buds the easiest. They contain a very high dose of HFCS; and to top it off, they are so readily available. **The advantage water has over sodas is the more you drink water with the reduction of sugary and greasy food, the less you will crave them.**

Why have we become used to drinking sodas with everything? Is it because it tastes that good, or is it because it comes with the value meal? Maybe it's because when you buy a fountain drink, the lever for water is so small that we just don't see it. Now, I'm not saying that you should never drink a soda. There are sodas without HFCS and I occasionally have one; but the irony is once you see the advantages of drinking water, you will see right through the cloudiness of sodas.

Drinking and Driving Don't Mix, but Drinking and Drive Do

The truth is any diet will work if you have the drive to stick with them. But drive doesn't just mean having the willpower to watch what you eat; it also means having the discipline to start an exercise program. If you watch the commercials for weight loss programs, there is always the fine print at the bottom on the screen that reads, "With exercise", along with the dreaded "individual results may vary." The Strategic Water Strike method is unique because it helps curb your appetite; but it is similar to all other diets because at some point in time you will have to incorporate exercise to continue to lose weight. So, the bad news is there is not a quick fix to healthy weight loss without exercising. **The good news is we can redefine the dirty little word called exercise and use it in a way that is compatible to your life.**

Exercise is just another word for movement. When I used to think of exercising, I used to think of the same old boring exercises and being at the gym. But now, I'm reminded of Jerry Rice the Pro Football Hall of Fame receiver. He once said that what helped him become a great receiver was working as a brick layer. He would have to catch bricks with his hands. That is not a traditional work out, but it was a great one.

So, exercise doesn't necessarily mean running a marathon at 6 AM or catching bricks. Try to redefine exercise as just finding 30 minutes a day to move around. It doesn't have to be all at one time. It can be 10 minutes here and five minutes there. Parking a little further when you are going shopping will kill at least a few minutes. Taking the stairs instead of the elevator will help. Even scheduling time to play with your kids will do the trick. Those ingenious little minds will figure out ways to keep you moving.

One key to starting and sticking with your exercise plan is to have many different activities. Redefine the word exercise by having many options you enjoy. Don't let it become boring and tedious. Don't think of it as exercise, but as staying active. Hey, here's an idea. Blow off the gym and go to the park or the beach. Don't tell yourself you need to do traditional boring exercises like the treadmill or sit-ups. Tell yourself, "I need to go outside and enjoy life!"

Most people don't enjoy doing the same thing everyday. So, mix it up. Find at least seven things you enjoy doing. On Monday go walking. On Tuesday go biking. On Wednesday jump rope. On Thursday wash the car. On Friday play with the kids. On Saturday mow the yard. On Sunday throw the Frisbee in the park. You get the point; do something different everyday to keep it interesting. Besides, your muscles need variety to help them grow. If you do the same routine every time, then you will keep your muscles from fulfilling their potential. The smaller muscles help support the bigger ones and you need to do various movements to work the smaller muscles. Varying your routine not only helps build muscles, it keeps your mind and your body interested.

Most plans to stay active fail because the exercise that was chosen is too strenuous. We don't feel like continuing because we are sore or too tired after the initial trial. The motivation is lost because we become discouraged and thus stop setting aside time to exercise. If you are just starting out, then schedule yourself to keep moving. But don't over do it. Make sure to leave yourself wanting more. For example, if you plan to start walking, then don't walk as far as you can on the first try. Try one slow trip around the block or just down the street. Make your first experience an easy one. Continue to make it easy until you want to increase your time and distance. Don't increase the difficulty because you feel you have to.

It's important to understand how exercising effects the goal to lose weight. Exercise builds muscles, but muscle is more compact than fat. So, don't only focus on the loss of weight; focus on the inches you lose around your waist. Do you want to fit in a smaller clothing size? Or do you want to just look and feel better? **Whatever the goal, you can actually trade being a little heavier for a small waist.** You might also want to build muscle because if you have cellulite, then it will look worse if you lose weight and don't build muscle. Exercising shapes your body, so choose activities that help augment the shape you want to be. Model your activities to the sports that have athletes whose body type you most admire. Each sport has it own body type. Although each athlete is different, there is something to be said about how a sport shapes the body.

Volleyball and softball players, sprinters, long distance runners, weight lifters, and swimmers all have a stereotypical body shape you can envision. Learn more about how those athletes prepare for their individual sports. Then, engage in the activities you enjoy and the exercises you think will shape your body to how you want it to look.

If you do enjoy going to the gym, that's perfectly fine, but take a break every once and a while to see what else is waiting for you. After all, we do need to stay active which doesn't mean just living in a gym. What would be the use of living longer if all we did were the things we don't enjoy? The most important key to keeping a steady routine is to make a plan and not vary from it, but vary with it.

Chalk It Up to Science Part II

Some doctors perform the surgery to staple your stomach to shrink it so you don't over eat. Ah, junk science strikes again. Well, not totally. Some patients actually do need this procedure, and it has been successful for them. For others, the procedure worked for awhile; then their stomach grew back to its original size. That's because the surgery doesn't teach you how to change your behavior or outlook on how food works for and against you. The Water Strike technique is meant to change behavior. It teaches you how to fish instead of just giving you one free meal at Red Lobster.

Did you know you can perform this procedure yourself? Yes, no needles. No doctors, No medical bills. And, it's all in the comfort of your own home. By using the Strategic Water Strike Method, you naturally shrink your stomach so to speak. With your stomach half full of water, it tells your appetite there is only a limited amount of seating. You effectively "water staple" your stomach every meal, but do it in a gentle way. Even if you wanted to eat more, your stomach will not be able to seat any more unwanted guests. One of the symptoms of the surgery was the patient could not physically eat much. If they did, it would come back up and they would still crave food.

Some people even go to the extreme procedure of wiring their teeth together to keep them from eating. But why go through that when you can easily control your hunger by drinking water? Does water really taste that bad?

Using the Water Strike Method curbs not only your appetite, but makes you feel less sluggish after a meal. If the Water Strike is used, then you shouldn't feel totally stuffed. You will feel full, but you shouldn't feel like your stomach is so packed that you can't move or be at the point that you have to unbuckle your belt; and you shouldn't experience stomach pain, which is a common feeling when your stomach is filled with just food.

I am not a scientist, but I am an expert on how I feel. Notice that I have been saying that you should feel this way or that way. The description on how you are feeling can help you learn to understand what may be happening in your situation. Is this next part junk science? It may or may not be. I am not a doctor, so take this next advice with a gain of salt.

It is important to listen to your body and notice how it reacts to certain foods. Most doctors don't stress that very much if at all. Really, they don't have time to micro-manage your health. Most doctors prescribe some medicines because they assume you have tried other remedies. (When was the last time you heard a doctor prescribing a glass of water without taking a pill?) Doctors might ask you if you are eating right and prefer a yes or no answer. They aren't going to ask you what you ate for breakfast every day for the past month. **They're not going to get that involved, but you should. It's your health we are talking about.** After all, it's inconvenient to go to the doctor's office. Most people don't like going, so doctors usually think you must really feel bad if you are there. Take some control in your life. If you are dissatisfied with your weight, then change what you are eating. If something doesn't feel right, then stop doing it and that includes eating.

If you are a little out of breath or having a hard time just breathing after a meal, it may be a sign your arteries are being clogged by excess fatty food. You may have eaten way over your allotted 65 grams of fat for the day. Most artery problems are created over time, but you should seek immediate medical attention if you have serious problems breathing. If you notice just a slight difficulty in breathing after eating, then the prescription could be a simple change in your diet. Remember what you ate and either limit it or don't eat it.

Listen to what your body is telling you. Look for signs that you are eating too much sodium. Most women can describe the feeling of being bloated during their menstrual cycle, but this feeling can also occur in men and women if too much sodium is consumed. If you do feel bloated or notice you have added a pound or two within a couple of days, then it might be sodium causing you to gain water weight. Limit the amount of salt you are consuming and you should see the loss of the extra weight in a few days.

Eating too much sodium can also cause a slight tingle or warm sensation in your body or slight pressure at the back of your head. Sodium can be linked to high blood pressure, but I am not sure if this sensation is your blood pressure rising. But try this: next time you eat something that is high in sodium, like a Frito Pie (which is notorious for being very high in sodium), see if you feel this sensation while eating. If you do, then remember it. Because the next time you get that same feeling while eating other foods, you are ingesting way too much sodium.

Most of us feel as though our stomachs stick out. But if you notice your belly is always feeling a bit heavy, it may mean you are eating too many fat filled foods. Try the Water Strike method with more fiber and less fat in your diet. The feeling of a heavy stomach should decrease. You will not only become a little lighter, but you will also feel the difference. Once you notice the difference, you will be able to tell when to cut back on heavier fat filled foods, like cheese for example.

The last example of noticing how your body reacts to food has to do with the debate about empty calories in unhealthy foods. The debate questions if the calories in healthy foods, like chicken and tuna, are the same as the calories in unhealthy food, like pizza. I don't know what the exact difference is, but there is big difference in the way they make you feel. The difference the calories make in energy levels is comparable to the feeling of being hydrated and being dehydrated. Once you start the Water Strike method, you should have more energy because you will be hydrated. It is not a life changing difference, but you will notice a difference. If you stop drinking water, you will notice a drop in energy levels; but don't take my word for it. Try your own experiment. Use the Water Strike method for a week and then stop. Remember how you feel without drinking water because you will feel the same if you eat just pizza as opposed to a good balanced meal; something in your energy level will be missing. **Doctors are there to help you, but next time you decide to get a check-up, start with your own personal physician…you.**

The Dietary Highway

The two most common questions regarding the dietary highway are "Won't I have to go to the bathroom every five minutes?" and "Where does the fat go?" We'll start with the most common question in regards to the Water Strike, and then address a common mystery concerning every diet.

The Water Strike method raises the obvious question. If you drink that much water, won't you have to go to the bathroom every five minutes? Yes and No. At first you will notice this technique will result in frequent trips to the bathroom; but after a while your body will adapt to the extra water intake. You will still have extra trips to the bathroom, but not constantly. You may not have to go the bathroom that often when you first try this method because you may be so dehydrated that your body might need the water. In that case, it may take a while to digest it; but in most cases you may have to make a few unexpected trips to the restroom. **Caution: the water will bring another unexpected occurrence.**

The additional water is a natural enema and will flush out (excuse the pun) toxins and waste. When most people have gotten this feeling before, they usually have had a bad experience to something they ate or remember it from the last virus they had. They remember it as a very bad experience, but it's not. It is just the water cleaning out your system, expect the unexpected until your system flushes out unwanted toxins and waste. Eventually your body will adjust to the extra water intake and you will feel better for it.

The mystery of where fat goes when weight is lost is not a major concern, but it raises an interesting question. How does fat leave the body? Well, the weight you lose will be disposed of through some obvious ways, but not exactly how you think. When calories are burned, fat cells are broken down, processed, and released mostly through urine. Some fat cells are broken down, processed, and released through sweat or evaporates. Fat is not released through fecal matter. Remember this if going frequently to the bathroom gets discouraging; weight loss is primarily release through urine, and water helps with that process.

Even though weight loss is not disposed of through fecal matter, it is important to keep total waste flowing out of your body. Water and fiber can be utilized to help with that process. Water and fiber flush out toxins and other waste. They are both high speed and low drag. Drinks that have high amounts sugar act like molasses and drag their feet on the dietary highway, and eating food with high fat content has the same effect.

It is important to know fiber is a great ally on the road to weight loss. Fiber will not only help keep you feeling full, it grabs all the bad cholesterol it can before it exits the body. Another word of caution: Your body may also take awhile to adjust to a higher fiber intake. Although apples, bran muffins, beans, and raisin bran cereals are high in fiber, great foods to fill your appetite, and help fight high cholesterol, they may get you running for the bathroom door. (Talk about exercising!) If you do have this experience, remember your body won't always react that way. It may take time for your body to adjust, but once it does it will make your trips to the bathroom a lot easier.

There is an old saying that an apple a day keeps the doctor away. I am not sure how accurate that is, but over all it is good advice. I don't know if I should be explaining this because I've never really seen it addressed. Maybe this is taboo, or maybe so obvious that I should not address the topic of actually using the bathroom. But the advantages of eating more fiber is it not only helps with the quickness, texture, and ease your food leaves your body and helps in dealing with hemorrhoids, it also removes fecal matter that is just lying in your intestines. No, it is not true 40 pounds of fecal matter was removed from either Elvis or John Wayne; but more fiber will help with the disposal of fecal matter, which means you will get an accurate measurement when you weigh yourself.

This is probably too obvious, but since I have already alluded to it, I will mention it anyway. Going to the bathroom shouldn't be a struggle. Do not force anything out of your body. You should be able to just sit and gently release waste. Sometimes you just have to sit for awhile until the waste is naturally released. If you are constantly having trouble releasing fecal matter, then it is because you do not have enough water and fiber in your diet. This is a giant clue because the Water Strike is about making healthy choices. If you are having trouble with the dietary highway, then you are not eating or drinking right. It is no secret that high fat foods can cause constipation; and it's no secret that healthier fiber filled food causes the exact opposite effect.

If you are still worried about the dietary highway being in high gear, you may try a banana for a snack. Almost everyone knows that bananas are high in potassium which is very good for you. But this secret assassin is useful in quickly killing your hunger and also pacing trips to the bathroom. However, too many in a day can bring the dietary highway to a screeching halt.

Try more water and food with higher fiber in your diet. Again, your body may take time to adjust; but your body will get used to it. Your body gets used to it because that's the way the body is supposed to function. It needs the extra water and fiber to clean out all the toxins and waste in your body.

Anyone Care for Second Breakfast?

Just like in the novel <u>The Lord of the Rings</u>, the hobbits got it right. A key to losing weight is to continue eating. But how could such a well intentioned idea of not eating derail your goal of losing weight. Well, when you skip meals or don't snack, your body slows down your metabolism and starts storing fat. It starts burning protein, which is reserved for building muscles, instead of burning carbohydrates that are used for energy. So, instead of losing weight you'll see little to no progress. If you feel hungry, then eat. Do not let hunger linger. It will slow down your metabolism.

Protein and carbohydrates are designed for two different tasks. Proteins build muscles, and carbohydrates are meant to be used as energy. If you just eat carbohydrates, you will not be utilizing their maximum potential to sustain fuel for your body, and vice versa for proteins. So, try to eat both proteins and carbohydrates together to optimize each role efficiently. If you don't eat them together, or don't eat at all, you will sabotage your diet and weight goals you worked so hard to achieve.

Think of it this way. If you were building a fire you would need firewood (proteins), and lighter fluid (carbohydrates). The firewood keeps a steady burn (metabolism), and the lighter fluid is used to start the fire and for keeping the fire burning when it starts to fade. If you don't use firewood (proteins), it's like starting a fire on concrete. You can use lighter fluid to start the fire, but the fire will burn out very quickly. It is equivalent to when kids eat too much sugar. They will start bouncing off the walls at first, but eventually they come crashing down. They weren't given any firewood (protein) to keep the fire burning.

In between your scheduled three meals a day, snack if you feel hungry. Eat foods that are mostly low in fat because eating fat ends up as body fat easier than carbohydrates or proteins. An ounce of fat gives you twice the amount of calories than an ounce of protein or carbohydrate. Try pretzels, Cheerios, Chex Mix, jerky, and fruits. Keep in mind the uses of proteins and carbohydrates; one is to fuel (carbohydrates) the body, and the other (protein) is to build it. Snacks that are high in starches are quickly converted to sugars, so it is important to balance proteins and carbohydrates. If you do snack on carbohydrates, but still feel like you are a little low on energy, then try some protein. You can even use some foods that are higher in fat, but are healthy for you like peanuts, almonds, string cheese, pistachios, and cashews. Peanut butter is great, but monitor the serving size because of the high fat content.

You may be pleasantly surprised to know it doesn't take much of a serving size to fight hunger between meals. For example, a serving size of ten pretzels has 110 calories. If you use the Water Strike method consistently, then a mere five pretzels can help curb your hunger until your next meal. And this will save you from eating the full amount of calories. Cashews are another example. They are higher in fat, but the serving size is 21 pieces. Cut the serving size and you will cut out half the fat. Ten pieces of cashews doesn't sound like it should be filling, but if you are using the Water Strike it will be reasonable. I am not forbidding you to eat a full serving size. The amount of how much weight you want to lose will determine how many calories to eat. The Water Strike gives you the option to choose how many calories to consume, and thus, how many pounds you lose.

Snack in between meals with carbohydrates and proteins to keep your blood sugar in check and your metabolism running. If you start to feel sleepy and lack energy in the middle of your work day or after a meal it may mean one of a few things.

It may mean you did not get enough sleep or you just ate too much, but it also may mean your blood sugar may be dropping and your metabolism is stopping which is caused by not eating enough carbohydrates. So, snack when you feel hunger or sleepy in the middle of the day.

It may also mean that you have ingested too many carbohydrates. In this case, you need to move to burn off the fuel provided by the carbohydrates and eat some protein. If you don't, then the extra carbohydrates will be stored as fat. Not a good thing.

How do you know what means what? Are you getting too many or too little carbohydrates? Well, you don't always know what the problem is until you try to remedy the situation to see what works. Now and then even doctors don't know exactly what's wrong. Occasionally, doctors don't know until they take many tests. Sometimes they prescribe one medicine to see if it works. If it doesn't, then they prescribe another. And that's not junk science. It just means every so often even in science it's a guessing game. Minimize the guessing in your diet by eating a balanced meal. Keep your body well fueled to achieve healthy weight loss.

But I Am an Addict!

"I have a sweet tooth and I love chocolate. I mean I would kill for chocolate!" Yes, some habits die hard. But we can't kill this habit nor do we want to. Most people think being on a diet means giving up the food we love and that is not necessarily true. We just have to apply the football coach's old saying when matched against a formidable opponent. "We can't stop them. We can only hope to contain them!"

So, how do we contain our weakness for sweets? First, don't eat sweets as a snack. Although it may be tempting to do, don't eat sweets in between meals. Make sure to snack between meals, but use items low in sugar. Eating sweets between meals will only increase your craving for them. This may result in having items loaded with sugar as your next meal.

Second, schedule three meals a day using the Water Strike method. Having regular scheduled meals prevents your body from panicking about your next meal. When your body panics, it not only slows down your metabolism, it creates chaos with blood sugar levels. Do not let hunger linger by skipping meals or not snacking. **If you let hunger linger, you will have an increase in craving your favorite sugary dessert.** The more you feel full with a balanced meal, the less sweets control your life.

Third, eat sweets only after you have used the Water Strike method and finished your meals. This will not only limit the craving for sweets, but also the amount of dessert you can eat. If you eat a balanced meal with the Water Strike method, you will be more likely to turn down sweets. If you don't turn down sweets, you will at least be able to turn down the offer of a bigger serving.

Shopping at a grocery store on an empty stomach can be a good metaphor for eating sweet before your meals. You tend to buy more when you are hungry. All reason to limit purchases goes out the window. But did you really need to buy donuts, Little Debbie cup cakes, and Twinkies? If you shop on a full stomach you can rationally decide which items you really need. Utilize this metaphor to stunt your craving for sweets. So, next time you are in your own kitchen shopping for sweets, do it on a full stomach.

Finally, do not stock pile sweets. Remember, dieting starts not at the point of eating, but at the point of purchase. Limit your purchases and don't keep them in view. Don't store them in convenient and easy to reach places. Out of sight: Out of mind. If you keep them right by the refrigerator, you will see and eat them every time you are hungry.

I don't recommend not buying any sweets because you do need a little flavor and sugar in your diet. Living life means enjoying the things you love and a balanced meal does include a little of everything.

Get In My Belly!

We are all familiar with a certain Austin Power's caricature that yells, "Get in my belly!" and we can empathize with him when we are starving. However, the Water Strike helps to lessen that empathy by curbing your hunger. An important point in this Strategy is to learn to eat for taste and not for hunger. This is a very important point to stress. Weight gain is caused by over eating, but part of the problem is mental. Because you are hungry, you believe a mass amount of food needs to be eaten to keep from starving; but that's not true. The body only needs a certain amount of calories. The Water Strike helps to rationally decide how many calories are needed. But since you enjoy food, you don't think twice about eating more than you should. The balance is to find a way to tame hunger and enjoy food.

This brings us to the concept of eating for taste. The Water Strike helps rule out thirst as hunger. This frees your mental state to enjoy eating, yet minimize calorie intake. **The eating for taste principle is simple; don't eat for hunger, eat for taste.** Try this experiment as a starting point to learn how to eat for taste. First, use the Water Strike method with one of your meals, and make sure you are pretty full. Second, choose something that is individually wrapped like a bite-size Snicker's or a Three Musketeer's bar, but make sure it is something you really like. Third, take a deep breath, and then put the candy in your mouth. Finally, exhale and chew slowly. You will notice the candy will not only taste great, but it will satisfy most of your craving. You may still want to eat a couple more, but you won't have the craving to eat the whole bag of candy. Using this technique will help you cut a lot of calories because you savor the small amount you eat. By eating less, you enjoy it more, and that's called eating for taste. It's about eating for quality and not for quantity.

The eating for taste principle isn't exclusively for food or dessert. Any drinks served with your meal also qualify. Just try to limit what you drink to eight ounces. It's important to apply this principle especially to drinks with high amounts of sugar. A good rule of thumb is to limit drinks that have more than 10 grams of sugar per serving. The bad news is that natural orange, grape, cranberry and apple juices all have over 20 grams of sugar; but because they are nutritious, you should drink them. The good news is using the eating for taste principle will allow you to be able to drink a couple of servings a day.

A good idea to get a couple of servings of juice and still limit sugar is to cut the serving size by putting ice cubes in your glass before you pour the juice. This way you can effectively water down your drink and not really notice because very cold drinks usually taste better (I like to do this instead of buying drinks with reduced sugar because I like to control the taste). Remember that a serving size of juice is only one eight ounce glass. So, if your glass is full of ice and you drink only four ounces of juice during each meal, you can still have one and a half to two servings of juice throughout your day.

If at this point you are thinking that one and a half to two servings of juice is not a lot, then you are not alone. I used to drink 16 to 20 ounces of orange juice during each meal. The point is to savor the amount you have. The Water Strike cures thirst first, so the instinct to gulp two to three servings during one meal is stopped. It forces you to rethink how many calories you actually need to drink. What seems like an unreasonable portion size will seem like a very reasonable amount if you understand the eating for taste principle; don't drink for thirst and don't eat for hunger, do it for the taste.

Summary

After reading this book, you should have learned a few very important things. First, the Water Strike will control hunger, keep you hydrated, and help you make healthier decisions for your diet. The Water Strike utilizes water to make you eat slowly, and that by default will help you realize you don't need to eat as much as you thought you did.

Second, listen carefully for all the subtle hints your body gives you. Whether it is the frequency of your bathroom breaks, energy levels, or hunger, your body is trying to tell you something and it usually involves water.

Third, you should have learned the eating for taste principles: drink water for thirst, and do not eat for hunger; eat and drink for taste.

In conclusion, with all you have read, I hope by doing even a few of the things I recommended that you will reach your ideal weight goals. If anything at least try the Water Strike method of two eight ounce glasses of water before eating any of your meals. It is equally important to schedule yourself to drink water just as you have scheduled yourself three meals a day. Remember, you can live without food for weeks, but without water you will die in a few short days. So, have drinking water as priority number one.

Again, there is really nothing new in this book. It is more of a reminder of all the things you were always told to do: count calories, exercise, eat right, and of course drink more water. But let me quickly recap each chapter:

1. **Eat a balanced meal**
2. **Make good choices**
3. **Use the Water Strike method: Drink two eight ounce glasses of water before every meal, and maybe a third afterwards**
4. **Count your calories**
5. **Don't eat foods with high doses of High Fructose Corn Syrup**
6. **Stay hydrated**
7. **Eat foods that you like**

8. **Don't drink sodas**
9. **Exercise**
10. **Beware of easy fixes, and listen to your body**
11. **Eat more fiber**
12. **Snack when you feel hungry**
13. **Enjoy the food you love, but don't do it on an empty stomach**
14. **Slow down to eat**

There you have it. Just like grandma and grandpa used to tell you. Well, not exactly. But remember, the most important part is to enhance your life by doing the things you love; and that always includes tasting the foods you love.

www.ingramcontent.com/pod-product-compliance
Lightning Source LLC
Chambersburg PA
CBHW060648290526
45793CB00001B/452